PEBBLES ON THE BEACH

Emma Higgins has eleven GCSEs, a GNVQ in health and social care, a BTEC national diploma in science and health studies and City and Guilds certificates in floristry. Pebbles on the Beach is her first published book, but she has already started to write a selection of poems for a children's book. Emma is twenty seven years old and currently lives in Ashford, Kent. She has been married for two years to her husband Steve who is a steel worker; they met nine years ago through a mutual friend. Also sharing their lives is their 18 month old Labrador, Holly.

PEBBLES ON THE BEACH

Emma Higgins

PEBBLES ON THE BEACH

Olympia Publishers
London

www.olympiapublishers.com
OLYMPIA PAPERBACK EDITION

A CIP catalogue record for this title is
available from the British Library.

ISBN: 978-1-905513-38-3

First Published in 2008

**Olympia Publishers
60 Cannon Street
London
EC4N 6NP**

Printed in Great Britain

Acknowledgements

This book is dedicated to my husband Steve who has given his all to help me through this ongoing nightmare. You are not only my husband but my closest friend. I am so privileged to have you in my life and I thank you for all the support you have given me through the years. Your belief in me has never wavered and your love for me has always stood strong. You have been there when I have had nobody else to turn to. I know I will get through this as long as I have you by my side and one day we will share in the happiness of life together. I owe you so much, I owe you my life. I'll end this by saying you are my world and I love you with all my heart, thank you babe for being you.

What is depression?

In one word, depression is an 'illness'. Many people don't see it as an illness they see it as just someone feeling down or sad. Every one of us at some stage will feel a bit low in our lives but these feelings tend to pass with time. Depression on the other hand is much more intense. It causes a chemical imbalance in the brain that does not only effect the individual mentally but also physically. The following is a list of some of the most common symptoms of depression and I have to admit it, I could tick every one of them at some point in my life.

- Difficulty concentrating

- Lack of sex drive

- Loss of desire for food

- Finding it hard to function at work/school

- Feeling useless and helpless

- Loss of energy and feeling tired a lot of the time

- Shutting yourself away from others often avoiding friends and family

- Physical aches and pains

- Very low self-esteem and self-confidence

- Relentless feeling of sadness

- Not getting enjoyment out of things that you once felt enjoyable

- Sleeping problems

- Unjustified feelings of blame and worthlessness

- Self-harm

- Contemplating suicide and death thoughts

Facts and figures

- At any one time, almost 10% of the general population are suffering from depression. (Paul Gilbert 1997)

- "It has been estimated that over 100 million people in the world today suffer from depression". (Paul Gilbert 1997)

- "One in four women and one in ten men will suffer a period of depression serious enough to require treatment through their lifetime". (Depression Alliance 1999)

- "Suicide threats should be taken seriously: about 70% of the 4000 suicides a year in Britain are among people suffering from depression and 15% of all those experiencing depression eventually commit suicide". (Sane – Depression and Manic Depression 1997)

- "Only 10% of people with depression consult their GP. Only 50% of those who consult are correctly diagnosed at the outset. Only 50% of those correctly diagnosed received medication at a therapeutic dose. Only 50% of those receiving medication at a therapeutic dose take their medication for more than twenty-eight days. Thus, only seven in one hundred patients with depression are effectively treated at the present time." (The Department of Health)

- "The illness depression is a serious medical condition with biological changes in the body and definite brain changes. This is why those who experience depression need professional help. The danger of this public perception is that people may leave it too long before seeking help – when depression has an excellent prognosis if recognised early and treated properly." Dr Raj Persaud – the Maudsley Hospital.

- The World Health Organisation estimates that by the year 2020, major depression will be second only to chronic heart disease as an international health burden (this is measured by its cause of death, disability, incapacity to work and the medical resources it uses).

- "More than 80% of people suffering from depression can be helped with appropriate treatment". (Depression Alliance 1999)

Famous people who have suffered from depression

* Artists (**Van Gogh, Georgia O'Keefe, Tracey Emin)**

* Actors (**Sarah Lancashire, Patsy Kensit)**

* Writers **(Ernest Hemingway, Sylvia Plath, JK Rowling)**

* Philosophers **(Nietzsche, Marx)**

* Politicians **(Winston Churchill – BBC's 'Greatest Briton' in a viewer poll)**

* Musicians **(Mel C)**

* Sportspeople **(Stan Collymore)**

* Comedians **(Ruby Wax, Caroline Aherne, Paul Merton, Stephen Fry).**

**Taken from Facts & More Info About Depression
www.alanpriest.com**

Introduction

Most people don't really understand depression unless they themselves or others close to them have been through it. It is not something you can just 'snap out of' which I have been told to do on several occasions. This is one of the reasons I decided to write this book as I found through personal experiences that some people's perception of this illness was very poor. I don't know whether it is down to lack of education on the subject, the unwillingness to learn about the illness or the big taboo that it's a mental health issue. I have found that some family members have been very negative about the fact that I have depression. They tend to shy away from the subject and pretend that everything is ok or worse still I have had things said to me that have pushed me even further down, but I have come to reside in the fact that it is THEM with the problem and not me. I feel that if I had a physical illness that people could see they would understand that I wasn't well but because it is inside and sometimes very well hidden it's hard for people to understand what is wrong. All I know is that depression has brought me so much sadness in my life and I have cried so many tears.

As I wrote this book I thought of all the people out there who are going through the same thing as me or are seeing someone they love going through this hell. I thought that with writing this book and sharing my feelings and emotions people would read it and if I could help just one person to realise that they are not alone there are many people going through the same thing then that would bring a smile to my face. I have no medical background so my whole book is based on what's in my heart and mind, I found it easier to write about my thoughts and feelings in the form of poems. I also have included sections of my diary which I have kept over the years. I really hope I can help you in some way.

Pebbles On The Beach...

I had felt depressed for as long as I could remember, the constant struggle just to live day by day. The feeling of worthlessness and loneliness in a world that just seemed to be passing me by. At first I tried to hide my illness from everyone. At the beginning I even tried to hide it from myself, not wanting to admit that anything was wrong. I'm not sure why, perhaps it was a feeling of shame or fear of the unknown. I was scared as I didn't know and didn't like the person I was becoming and I didn't understand why I couldn't just pick myself up again. The occasional 'off' days seemed to get more and more frequent, then before I knew it everyday was an 'off' day and it had taken over my life completely.

As the years went on I saw depression as my enemy, every day was a fight just to cope with the smallest of tasks. I felt that I was in a constant battle to get better but the worse thing was what I was battling against had made me so weak both mentally and physically that I would sometimes feel that I was fighting a losing fight.

I can't put my finger on when my depression started. It just seemed to creep up on me without my realising. I remember feeling 'down' more often than other people seemed to be when I was younger but I thought that was just my personality. As I went into my teens I began to have a very volatile relationship with my mum and at this stage this is when things for me progressively got worse.

I was fifteen when I started to self-harm, I remember it well. I had recently found out that my granddad had cancer. I was very close to my granddad and the news hit me hard. I had never lost anyone close to me before and I found I just couldn't deal with it. One lunch time at school I walked to nearby woods. I just sat and cried and as I cried I noticed a bit of old glass stuck in the mud next to me. I don't know what came over me but I took it, cleaned it on my jumper and then just started cutting my wrists, it didn't hurt at first as I was too upset to feel the pain but when the blood started to run down my arms the pain and reality stepped in and I couldn't believe what I had done, but strangely I felt an unbelievable sense of calm come over me. Since that day I have self-harmed many times; it was my way of punishing myself with not being able to cope with life and to get all my hurt and anger out. I'm not proud of it; in fact I hated myself even more after I had done it because I felt so weak. A lot of people talk of control when they self-harm and I feel that's what it partly was for me. Depression seemed to have taken over control of my life and cutting myself was my way of getting that control back, but as I look back at it now, I wasn't in control, it made me feel as if I was, but why would I really choose to cut myself? It's just so scary to think how much power your mind can have over you. I'm pleased to say that I haven't self-harmed for over two years. Don't get me wrong there are times when things get on top of me and the urge to do so is unbearable but I just think to myself, I don't want anymore ugly scars on my body reminding me of the past, in the future I don't want my kids to ask me what the marks on my arms are and the thought of that and the support from my husband has made me realise I just don't need or have to do that any more.

After school I went on to college with all the same feelings I had grown used to living with, I just accepted this was how I felt, this was how I was always going to feel so I just had to get on with it. I got really good at this stage at putting on a front and basically living my life as two different people. At college I was always the life and soul of the class, always the one to crack the jokes and make everyone laugh but inside I was hiding the 'real' me. I would go home, cry myself to sleep, so messed up in my own world, and when I was really low I would cut myself, I wouldn't tell anyone I would just hide it with long sleeves or bangles around my wrist and I would put back that smile and make believe that everything was alright again. This carried on throughout the two years of college and into my next job after that.

In 2000 I started my first full time job. I worked in the maternity ward at my local hospital. It felt a bit daunting at first as there was so much to learn and take in but I eventually got my head around it and came to really enjoy it. My depression was still there but with so much to occupy my mind and not wanting anyone that I met to know that I was ill I carried on hiding it. It became like a dark secret I was ashamed of the person that I really was and it was easier to act out the person I wanted to be, that way I didn't have to answer difficult questions and I wouldn't have to face rejection or prejudice.

After about a year in my job the mask that I was wearing day in and day out was starting to wear thin. The feelings of loneliness and isolation and constant sadness were so overwhelming and I finally admitted to myself that I just couldn't cope anymore. At this stage the self-harm was getting worse but as I was working I found ways of hiding it. I would cut my stomach and legs instead of my arms so no one would see. Eating had also became a problem, I found that I couldn't eat in front of people anymore, I'm not sure why, I just started to feel that everyone was looking at me and judging me and I became very self-conscious. At lunch times while the rest of the staff would eat in the staff room I found that I would make an excuse to be somewhere else. I would often end up in the public toilets at the front of the hospital where I would sit in a cubicle and pick at my lunch. I know that was the most disgusting place to be, but for me it was the only place I felt comfortable. No one could see me and no one could judge me so it made me feel safe.

My eating habit slowly got worse and worse, my lunch times spent in the toilets became an everyday occurrence but now I felt guilty after eating. I felt fat and I had an overpowering need to get out of myself what I had just put in, that's when I started to make myself sick. I can't explain to you the way I felt inside after I had for example just eaten a sandwich. I hated myself for being so weak and giving in to food, I hated myself for not being strong enough to resist. I would make myself sick after everything that touched my lips. It became an everyday routine; just something I would do, not just after every meal but also if I was to have a glass of squash then that would need to come up too. I would not be able to relax until I had been sick, again like the self-harm this became my secret that I hid from everyone.

At home things weren't any better I was still having a hostile relationship with my mum with arguments being a day to day way of communication. Other things I noticed were when I was out I felt that everyone was looking at me and sometimes I felt that they were laughing at what a mess I had became. Although I still wore my makeup and dressed nicely I was convinced people could see the absolute failure that stood before them. This became worse and worse, I would walk into a shop and if anyone looked at me I would walk straight out again. I started to suffer from really bad panic attacks both at work and at home, sometimes they would be manageable because I learnt how to breath through them but other times my heart would beat so hard and so fast I would feel that it was going to burst through my chest, at these times I would just hid away from people either in a toilet or in my bedroom until the feeling passed. Getting on a bus was a nightmare because again I felt all eyes were on me thinking what a loser I was, this got so bad that I eventually got a taxi everywhere which cost me a fortune but I didn't care because at least it meant I only had to face one person instead of a whole bus load. Going out then went down to the bear minimum; I wouldn't go into town on my own anymore I would just use the taxi to get to and from work.

I found work increasingly getting harder, along with being weak from my eating disorder I was mentally exhausted from pretending to be someone that I wasn't, living my life as a lie. I was getting sick of putting on this 'happy' act to please other people; it was getting harder with every day. Working in an hospital you are suppose to help other people and make them better which I did every single day but sometimes I just felt like screaming 'help me' I really wanted someone to help me to get better and get me out of this hell in which I was living.

In September 2001 I finally gave in to myself and admitted that I had a problem. Up until now the only person to know that I was ill was my partner Steve. I went to see my doctor and explained how I was feeling and he put me on medication, which in turn made me feel even more disappointed in myself for not coping. I started to cut myself more and more because I didn't know of any other way to cope with all my mixed up feelings that ranged from sadness to anger and hate. I was walking around like a zombie at work so the only thing for me to do was to tell my manager about the situation and explain that I just couldn't cope on a day to day basis anymore. She was really helpful and understanding, it just felt like such a relief to get it all out into the open. She phoned another ward in the hospital and managed to get a psychiatrist to come and see me. After a long discussion everyone decided that I needed some time off of work.

Once off of work my doctor decided to double the dose of medication I was on, I was also referred to and started seeing a psychiatrist. He went through everything with me and tried his best to help but I just felt that he wasn't understanding how I was really feeling. I wasn't understanding how I was feeling so how was anyone else going to? After about three weeks of seeing him for consultations my mood was not lifting and I started to feel that the only way out would be for me to just end it all and commit suicide. I attempted this twice but I thank God now that I didn't succeed. I discussed my feelings with my psychiatrist and he agreed that the tablets that I was on had not done anything to raise my mood. I was referred back to my doctor who then changed my medication in a bid to help sort me out. I carried on with my consultations with my psychiatrist he gave me tasks to do, for example, go into town on the bus. He also asked me to keep a diary of all my thoughts and feelings and that we would talk about and come up with solutions to different situations I had faced and wrote about each week. I must say that writing my thoughts and feelings down did help me to start to deal with my depression.

After about eight weeks I managed to get myself back to work, the new medication I was on had started to help. I had stopped cutting myself for a while and over the course of time making myself sick eventually stopped. I even felt well enough to stop seeing my psychiatrist. I was a hundred per cent better than I was but I still wasn't a hundred per cent in myself if you know what I mean. I was back to how I felt at college, I would feel so down and so isolated in myself but again I tried to put this to the back of my mind and say to myself that was just 'me'. Again I started faking my smiles and pretending that I was okay and that I had got through this but all I was doing was lying to others but most of all, I was lying to myself.

Steve and I decided to get a house together in the summer of 2002. We finally moved in December 2002. Our first Christmas together that year was the best I had ever had, although the house was a mess and we didn't have much money it was just nice being together. I think I thought or I hoped that all my problems would disappear as soon as we moved in together. I was wrong. I didn't have the arguments that I used to have with my mum anymore, but my head was still so messed up. I was okay if I kept myself busy with work or with decorating the house but as soon as I had time to think about things I would fall apart. Steve is in a job where he has to work away a lot of the time so I had a lot of long lonely days and nights when all I could do was think.

My nightmares got worse. I have a recurring dream that I have had since I was about fifteen. I dream that I am in this room or I call it a 'cell', the floor, ceiling and walls are all concrete, there are no windows or doors so there is no way out. I am sitting in the middle of this room, I look up and I see the ceiling slowly coming down on me and the walls are slowly closing in on me. The feeling of absolute terror and panic are so overwhelming as it always seems so real. I always end up screaming and I am often out of my bed either lying on the floor with my fingers wedged under the door or I'm by the window. I never usually wake on my own, Steve ends up having to shake me out of it. On one occasion when Steve was working away, I had one and of course no one was there to wake me up and bring me around and I ended up putting my hand through my bedroom window. I woke in complete shock as my hand was pouring with blood. The next day I went to the doctor's and he put me on different antidepressants. I still to this day have those dreams. They are less frequent but still as frightening.

Over the following four years depression still stayed with me but I learnt to cope with it. I learnt that everyday I had to really push myself to achieve the smallest of things. I would feel tearful and down ninety per cent of the time and angry and hateful the other ten per cent. I could deal with the tearfulness but I hated myself so much when all the hate and anger came out because I used to take it all out on Steve, I would shout at him for the smallest of things and I would get so frustrated with things that were so insignificant. I guess it's true what they say, that you take things out on the people that are nearest and dearest to you and that was the case. Steve is everything to me, he has always been there for me through this illness and he understands me like no one else ever could. We got married on the twenty fourth of July 2005 and that was the happiest day of my life.

Shortly after the wedding though things for me started to get increasingly worse again I think it was because my feelings were put aside while I had so much to think about with the wedding that when it was all over they all came back with a bang. I should have taken note of the warning signs and got myself sorted sooner rather than later but I chose to ignore them, to put them to the back of my mind and not want to believe that I was going down again. I have learnt that depression is much like a rollercoaster. You never know what is around the corner or how deep the drop will be, whether you'll come straight back up again or whether you'll carry on falling.

I was now on my fourth different type of antidepressant and they didn't seem to be working very well but then again how was I to know how I would feel if I stopped taking them? Would I feel any worse? I wasn't prepared to find out so I carried on taking them. With work I just coped, I went, did my job and came home. I felt if I could just cope with everyday tasks I would be okay. It seemed that everyday I would function on autopilot.

Slowly though I found going into work increasingly getting harder, sometimes I would cry for hours before my shifts because I really couldn't face going in and when I came home I would cry again. Other times Steve would have to physically force me to walk through the door and more and more often I would start to make up excuses as to why I needed a day off. On my days off I found it so hard to get out of bed I was just so tired all the time. I would maybe come down stairs for a packet of crisps or so and then go back to bed, I found it easier that way as it made the long days shorter. I would dread the next time that I was to work, counting down days, hours and minutes until I had to walk through the door. When in work people would talk to me and I would smile and say that everything was okay but I found that I would go into a dream world most of the time, I would hear people laughing and joking, they would be sitting right next to me but it would all sound so muffled and far away. I could be sitting in the crowed staff room with people all around me yet I would feel so alone.

I had never felt this low before, nothing made me happy, nothing I did gave me a break from how I was feeling. I eventually lost the ability to lie to people about how I felt, I couldn't even pretend to smile and be happy. It felt that I had nothing left inside me I was totally dead within. It all came to a head on the fourteenth of November 2005. I was on an early shift at work, in handover I kept thinking to myself that I just couldn't do this anymore. I went out onto the ward and I just felt like I was going to fall to pieces. Again as I had experienced before I went into some sort of daze. Everything seemed to be a million miles away, people were talking and the usual hustle and bustle of the ward was happening but it felt like I wasn't there, for a moment it actually felt as though I had died and left my body because I could see everyone rushing around me and I was watching people getting on with their daily tasks but I seemed to be caught in slow motion unable to move, unable to talk, unable to exist. Suddenly the silence was broken by a midwife tapping me on the shoulder and asking me to help a mother feed her baby. Again on autopilot and still in my dream state I walked to the room and instead of doing what I had done for over ten years, smiling and making small talk and pretending that everything was alright, I took her baby, sat down and fed it. I was thinking to myself that I needed to be talking to this mum that I was coming across so rude but how ever much I tried, no words would come out. I finished feeding her baby, I said goodbye and left the room. As I closed the door and walked onto the corridor I remember it looked so long, again everything seemed so far away, I could hear all the voices in the background, what they were saying I couldn't comprehend, the buzzers were going off and people were rushing around as I used to do. I carried walking along the corridor which seemed to go on for miles, people would pass me sometimes as if I was invisible other times just give me a sideward glance. I reached the staff room which seemed like I had been walking for hours, I picked up my bag and I left, I walked out of the hospital and I never went back.

I'm not sure whether I had some sort of breakdown but the months that followed were my darkest months ever. I was a complete and utter mess. I would wake up in the morning with my alarm clock and I hated the fact that I had even woke up at all. I would literally have to drag myself down the stairs. Once downstairs I couldn't face looking in the mirror anymore to do my makeup because I hated the person staring back at me. So I didn't bother. I didn't bother brushing my hair and there were some days when I couldn't even face washing. I wouldn't get dressed. I would stay in my pyjamas. I would go into the living room and sit on the settee, the television would then be switched on and there I would stay for the rest of the day. I would flick from channel to channel trying to find something that would take my mind off of what I was feeling. I would try to watch comedy sketches to try and see if that would help but nothing worked. I would sit for hour after hour just staring at the screen not able to take anything in, it finally felt like I had given up, it felt like there was nothing left in me any more. I just felt dead.

Other days would be a mixture of staring at the television and going back to bed. They were what I called the 'good' days. The 'bad' days were something completely different. I would get up, turn the television on but instead of just sitting there and watching the television I would slowly feel the tension and frustration building up inside of me like a kettle coming up to boil. As the tension and stress was getting worse I found that I would start rocking. I remember thinking to myself I really have gone mad now. I would rock for hours on end. Sometimes crying, other times in silence. Eventually it felt uncomfortable and I used to feel frustrated when I stopped rocking, like the rocking was the 'normal' thing to do. Other times I would get up and I would have a line in my head like 'I can't cope anymore' or 'nobody understands' or 'I hate myself' and I would walk around my kitchen and keep saying the same line over and over again out loud. Sometimes this would last for hours, other times it would go on all day.

I hated myself so much, I hated the utter failure that I had become. When I did on the off chance look into the mirror I remember feeling so disgusted with myself. The fact that I had let the depression win and reduce me to this total mess of a person made me feel like such a useless and pathetic being. Nothing made sense anymore I felt like a prisoner in my own home but most of all a prisoner in my own head. I used to keep all my curtains drawn and the doors locked because I did have a tiny bit of self respect left, that's about all I had left. I didn't want my friends and family to see me like that and to be honest I think if anybody saw me that way they would have insisted that I went into hospital. The only person to see the true extent of how I was, was Steve. Also I feel I hid it from my family because some of them had already told me about how they felt towards my depression and I couldn't handle any spiteful comments or rejection with the way I was feeling at the time I think it would have pushed me over the edge. So I just carried on, I remember thinking to myself you have to go down before you get back up again and I can hand on heart say that I was at rock bottom. There was no way I could have gone any further down so with that in mind that gave me the encouragement to think that I would get through this, there was only one way to go now and that was up. It wasn't easy, my life revolved around sitting in my pyjamas, rocking, crying and hating myself for months and months.

My first turning point was I set myself a goal so that every day when I got out of bed I would go straight into the shower get out, get dressed and put on makeup. Even the small thing about putting on makeup made me feel that little bit more human. The next task that I set was with the television I would tell myself after the shower I would watch television for one hour. After that hour I would turn it off and get on with some housework. This really started to work well, the curtains were opened eventually and the door was unlocked and after about six months I decided one day to go up the town on my own on the bus. Don't get me wrong I felt sick with anxiety, what if I have a panic attack? What if people stare at me? What if people know what a loser I was? All these questions passed through my head but then other questions passed through, Do I really want to live my life hiding away from the world? Do I want this depression to win? And with these questions my mind was made up. I grabbed my coat, took a deep breath and went. I made sure I made this a regular occurrence, although sometimes I didn't feel like it

I would push myself because I didn't want to slip back down. Slowly I started to get myself back on track and that leaves me with where I am today.

After a long struggle with a lot of withdrawal symptoms including the shakes, dizziness and nausea I managed to get myself off my antidepressants which I am very proud of. I know I have been off of them before but this time I am determined to stay off them. Depression has made me a stronger person in some ways but in others it has taken its toll on me. I feel stronger because I managed to beat it, I haven't forgot about my rollercoster theory where we don't know what is around the corner but I feel that I went down a very big drop and I managed to get back up again so I feel if there are anymore drops in my life to face then I will be much more able to deal with them knowing that I have been there before. I really wish that the rollercoster would stop and that I could just get off but it won't because that is life, life is just one big ride with twists and turns and some bumps on the way. On the down side I feel loss, I feel that depression has stolen so many years of my life that can't ever be replaced. I also feel like I've let myself and other people down. I have felt this way ever since I walked out on my job. I used to love my job it gave me a sense of purpose it was nice to know that people needed me and that I could help them, I haven't got that anymore so in a way that feels like another loss. I think the reason I haven't gone back into a job is because I am so scared of going back down again. I'm not ruling out getting a job in the future I'm just not at that stage at the moment. It has also left me with low self-esteem and lack of confidence which hopefully with time I will be able to build on. In the past couple of years I have also started to suffer from the checking form of obsessive compulsive disorder which takes over a lot of my time each day. But I can deal with these things they are all manageable when I get fed up or down with them I make myself remember what I was like and how much better I am now and nothing could ever compare to going back down there again. I know that depression will always be a part of me. I feel it will stay with me for the rest of my life but the way I have come to deal with it is to always say to myself that I need to stay in control and as long as I have that control I won't fall down. There are many times when I still have my 'off' days but every time I have them I push myself, I push myself to go out and I push myself to just get on with life because as soon as you lose that oomph to do so there is always a chance that depression could take back that control. When I do get down Steve makes me feel positive. He reminds me of all the good times we have got to look forward to, most of all having children of our own. When he talks about that I feel that maybe I have got a purpose in this life. I'd love to be a mum one day, I know I will get there I know it'll be hard and that there will be some setbacks but I am determined to make it. With writing this book I found that it has helped me to deal with my thoughts and feelings and even some of my fears. I feel that it has made me a stronger person for it, I just hope it can help you in some way. Think what you want in life, think of the happiness you want to find, and push yourself, set yourself realistic goals and tasks and keep working at them and if you have setbacks or bumps in the road don't let it stop you. Work even harder. I didn't used to believe it but now I know that there is so much to live for, every moment is precious you might not see it now but that might be because that happiness you are searching for is just around the next corner.

I decided to call my book 'pebbles on the beach' because that is how I see life. Anyone of us could be that pebble lying on the sunny beach when suddenly without warning a big wave could come along and drag us out to sea. Some of us won't get dragged in very far by the sea and will eventually get back out again onto dry land. Others will go in that little bit further and will need an extra bit of help to get out again. And others will be engulfed by the huge black ocean unable to breath and some may even drown. As I have said before through my depression I have had to deal with some really negative responses from people and even some really cruel remarks but I want these people to know that anyone of us at any time could get dragged under by the waves of depression so we shouldn't judge other people by what we don't understand.

<u>Depression</u>

D is for the despair that I feel every day

E is for the emptiness that doesn't go
away

P is for the pain that I feel deep inside

R is for the regret of the hurt I've had
to hide

E is for my eyes which have cried so
many tears

S is for the sorrow which has plagued
me through the years

S is for the sadness of the dreams I've
left behind

I is for in my heart the happiness I
hope to find

O is for my other self that's happy,
content and free

N is for this nightmare that has taken
over me.

This big world

I feel so small in this big world
So insignificant in size
If I were to disappear tomorrow
No one would recognize

I feel like screaming at the top of my
     voice
Wanting someone just to hear
But scream and scream as loud as I can
My screams just disappear

I feel so tiny in this huge earth
I've nothing left to give
I seem to have no purpose in life
Every day I wake to just live

I want someone to take my hand
And make everything alright
To guide me to a happy place
From the darkness into the light

I've known that my granddad has had cancer for about six months now. It tore my world apart when I found out as I am very close to him and the thought that I'm going to be losing him soon is too much to take in. My mum thought it best that he didn't know what was wrong with him and in a way I agree with her because finding out that would break his heart but on the other hand it is killing me lying to him and pretending that every thing is alright. At the moment he is ok as he doesn't have much pain and he is still getting on with

his day to day tasks. I just don't know how I
will cope when he gets worse.

<u>June 1995</u>

Things at home are really bad at the moment, I know my mum is upset about granddad but so am I. There are times when I just want her to sit down and talk to me about it and give me a hug because I am so scared, I have never lost anyone close to me before and it is tearing me apart seeing him just slowly dying knowing there is nothing I can do to help him.

I skipped school today and went to a woods nearby, I sat and for the first time since finding out that I would lose my granddad I cried, but I couldn't stop crying I just felt so useless and alone, I couldn't imagine life without him.

I saw a piece of broken glass nearby and I don't know what came over me but I just started cutting my wrists with it. I kept cutting until I couldn't take the pain anymore. I threw the glass down and I couldn't believe what I had just done but strangely I felt much calmer and able to cope. I cleaned myself up and hid it from everyone.

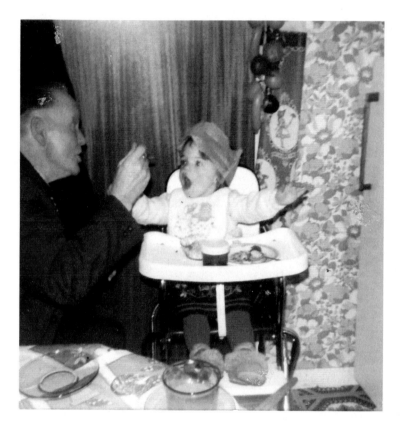

Me with my Granddad when I was about two.

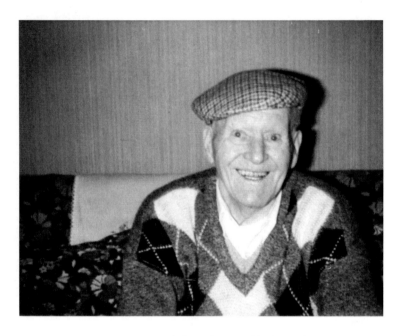

My much loved Granddad.

<u>April 1996</u>

Granddad is really bad at the moment; he keeps having falls and he is now on morphine to help with the pain he is in. My mum cooks him his dinner and when I get home from school we walk the twenty minute walk to his house. I always dread what we will find when we get there I always take a deep breath before we go through the door and pray that he's alright.

Today he had really bad pains in his stomach. I looked at him and lied, which I hate myself for. I said I had got a stomach ache too and that it must have been the strawberries we ate yesterday. For a split second I hoped that he'd believe me but I could see in his eyes he knew it was something more.

I haven't been coping well lately I have been skipping school a lot and the self-harm has got worse as I feel it's my only way to deal with things. I just can't handle the fact he is dying and is in so much pain. I just pray every night that he would go in his sleep and then he wouldn't have to suffer anymore.

November 1996

Granddad has had to go into hospital now as his pain can't be controlled from home anymore. He has lost a lot weight and they are pumping him with so much morphine, he is hallucinating and he doesn't really know who anyone is. Today I was sitting with him and he thought he could see a rat run across the floor, then he started re-living the war and he saw all the planes flying over.

<u>October 21st 1996</u>

My granddad died last night at 6pm, I'm glad

his pain is over but life will never be the same

again without him.

Wish upon a star

When you wish upon a star, your
      dreams come true
When I was a little girl this is what I
      was told to do.
I remember searching the sky for the
      brightest star
And thinking to myself how will my
      wish travel that far?

I used to close my eyes and think of my
      biggest dream
A new Barbie, a new bike or some
      strawberry ice cream.
A puppy would be nice, or maybe a
      rabbit instead
I'd love it to snow tonight while I'm
      tucked up in my bed.

But now I only have one dream, but
      however much I try
I can never find my star as I search the
      midnight sky

When I was little the stars were so
bright
Now all I see is darkness as the day
turns to night

All I dream is to be happy with no more
tears
But I've wished the same wish for years
and years
I guess my wishing star has fallen out of
the sky
Because I'm still sitting down here
dreaming, but still I cry.

The pain within

The first cut stings but that soon
     disappears
The second and the third are awash
     with tears.

The fourth and the fifth this is how I
     survive
As the blood starts to weep, I know I'm
     alive.

Each cut is deeper than the one before
By the fourteenth and the fifteenth it
     begins to get sore.

But I carry on cutting until the pain
     grows too much
My skin is so tender I can barely touch.

The pain on the outside can't compare
     to within
The never ending battle I can never win.

It's my way of releasing all the hurt
  inside
To see the blood flow I know I've not
  died

I mop up the blood and tidy away
My punishment is over until another
  day

January 2001

I remember having bad dreams last night, I can't remember what they were about but I kept waking up. I got to work and brought a sandwich I had to go and sit in the toilet and eat it though, I've been doing this for the past two days because I can't eat in front of people anymore and anyway, whenever I eat now I always end up nearly bringing it up again and I don't want people to see me like that. I keep having panic attacks lately, about three or four a day but today I really didn't feel well, it started off with the shortness of breath, the really strong heart beat and the shaky feeling but this time it lasted the whole of my shift and it just wouldn't go away. It's now 11.15pm and I'm just lying in my bed thinking I must be the most worthless person in the world, I feel I have no part to play in life and most of all I just feel so lonely.

September 2001

I went to the doctor's after work today and he has put me on antidepressants, I didn't want it to come to this. I just hope they're going to help because I really can't cope any longer

I felt a bit better today after last night, I can't explain what happened to me because I don't even know myself. I'd had a nice surprise from my boyfriend, he had brought me a bunch of flowers which really cheered me up but as soon as I walked through my door I just felt all stressed and tense again. I went to my room and I really just wanted to get into bed and go to sleep but I couldn't. I got one of my pieces of broken glass out which I keep hidden in my drawer and I just needed to get my frustration out, by this time I was naked and standing in front of my mirror, I looked at my reflection and I hated everything about what I saw. I started scratching my arms and legs with my nails then I looked at my stomach and started cutting it again, I can't explain what was going through my head because it was blank, no feelings, no thoughts just frustration and hate for myself. I kept cutting until I couldn't take the pain anymore, then I felt better. I saw another psychiatrist today he seemed to think he could help me but to be honest I really think I am beyond help, maybe he can, what can I lose?

The stranger in the window

I look out of my window
And I'm shocked to see
I didn't know anyone was there
But there's someone staring back at me

She is standing there naked
With her head bowed low
I've seen her somewhere before
It's a girl I feel I know

She looks up to face me
I give her a smile
She's shaking all over
She's been standing there a while

I see a tear run down her check
Her eyes are red and sore
She looks like she's given up on life
Like she just can't take anymore

I see the scars on her body
Each showing a pain she's had to hide

But no one can see the true hurt
The biggest scars are hidden inside

She's staring at me
Longing for a helping hand
She tries so hard to tell people
But no one seems to understand

She then falls to the floor in a heap
Her sobs ring through my ears
I ask her how long she's felt like this
 She says she's felt this way for years

I reach to hold her hand
But it's stopped by the window pane
It's getting colder and colder outside
And now it's started to rain

I'm trying so hard to see her
But the rain is blurring my view
I can see her in the distance
I just don't know what to do

Something warm hits my leg
I realise it's a tear

I wipe my eyes on my hands
And the window seems to clear

She appears again as clear as ever
Sitting right in front of me
She looks me straight in the eye
And for the first time I can see

I know who this girl is
I remember how she used to be
There's no window, but a mirror
It's a reflection... it's me.

Mind games

I can't explain what is going on inside
my head

Because I don't even know.

Sometimes it's filled with so much I feel
it could explode

But other days my mind is just blank.

When I'm down it is like a tape recorder
it plays me back all the hurtful
things people have said to me
over and over again.

And on the off chance when I'm happy
It reminds me to be sad.

I wish sometimes I could swap with
someone for just one day to make
them understand how it feels.

But then being free of it for just a while
I know I would never ever want it back.

You wouldn't think that your mind
        could stop you from doing day to
        day tasks, but it can.

You wouldn't think that your mind
        could have so much control over
        you that it makes you want to just
        give up

But it does.

Ticking of the clock

My alarm clock rings out
But I've barely gone to bed
I reach to turn it off
And pull the covers over my head

I often wish that I didn't wake
And have to face the day
That in my dreams I dreamt at night
I would softly drift away

I listen as the clock softly ticks
As the hand moves slowly by
Life is like a ticking clock
When one day your battery will die

A minute, an hour
A week, a year
Time goes by so quickly
But I'm still frozen here.

The never ending fight

This feels like I am fighting
A never ending fight
It starts early in the morning
And goes deep into the night

I take two steps forward
But get pushed back another four
I walk towards the open window
But find a closed door

Sometimes I hear the birds sing
Maybe things aren't as bad as they seem
The sun shines so brightly
But I wake, It was just a dream

I look into the mirror
And what stares back at me
Is a person I don't really know
Someone I forgot to be

I feel that I am just a shell
Who's dead and cold inside
I walk around just in a dream
But deep within I've died.

January 2002

I felt really down today. I'd been at work this morning and everything is starting to get on top of me again. I picked up my three months' supply of antidepressants from the chemist. I already had a pack of painkillers in my bag and I brought another pack in the local shop. I walked to a lake nearby and I sat down. I just thought, "this is it, I am going to kill myself I have just had enough of living my life like this." As I sat at the lake I watched people walk by, I saw people with children laughing and playing, I saw couples walk past hand in hand with their whole future ahead of them, I just thought to myself, "if depression is all I've got to look forward to, if this is my only future then what is the point." I started taking the tablets until I felt a bit distant but then the weak, scared side of me set in and I found I couldn't go through with it. I feel like such a failure I can't seem to do anything right, I can't even do the smallest of things like take a couple of tablets. I hate myself so much, I just want to die.

<u>February 2002</u>

I woke up this morning and I felt that I just couldn't go on anymore. I often wake up feeling like this but today the feeling was so strong I just didn't have any control over it. Mum was at home and I had the day off. I asked for a bath and I had the usual confrontation but today it was different I just didn't care anymore I didn't even have the strength to argue back.

I ran my bath and got in and then I had the most overwhelming feeling to just end it all, I felt that I would be so much better off dead. I hate my life and every thing about my life and I just feel I am not ever going to get over this.

I slid under the water and instead of holding my breath I closed my mouth and breathed the water in through my nose. I remember thinking to myself, if I do this long enough my lungs will fill up with water and I will eventually drown. I kept doing it over and over again, my chest was getting tighter and I was starting to become really dizzy and sick. Every time I went under it seemed like I was going into another world, everything became muffled and I seemed to just relax. It felt like this was my time, I wasn't scared I felt so focused on what I was doing and for the first time in ages I felt calm.

Just as my head was getting really faint my mum started banging on the door for me to hurry up. I snapped out of the state I was in immediately. It felt like I had been dropped down to earth again with a bang. I feel that if my mum hadn't knocked on the door I would be dead now because the feeling that I had was a feeling I have never felt before, I was just so peaceful and free.

I slowly got out of the bath and I felt terrible, I laid on my bed for a while and the room just spun and my head was hurting so much. I just needed to get out of the house, so I put my coat on and walked round the corner to my sister-in-law's house. She knew about my depression but she didn't know quite how bad it was. I told her about my headache which by now was unbearable. She had two young children and she couldn't drive so there wasn't much she could do for me. I had taken some painkillers but they weren't working one bit. In the end I was crying out in pain. But I still didn't admit to her what I had done. I decided I needed to get a taxi to the hospital. The taxi journey was a complete blur, the pain in my head was unbearable. The taxi driver had to help me into A & E as I was so bad. They asked me loads of questions but I found I couldn't tell them what I had tried to do as I felt ashamed not for the fact that I had tried to commit suicide but for the fact I hadn't been strong enough to carry it through. I laid on the bed and I can honestly say I have never felt pain like that before in my life. They gave me some stronger pain killers but again they didn't help. Eventually I was sent for a brain scan because by this time I was now rolling around on the bed and had started being sick. Luckily the brain scan come back ok, by now I had been in hospital about eight hours and my head ache was starting to ease. Steve came and picked me up from the hospital after he had finished work, I couldn't even bring myself to tell him what I had done. I got back home it was like I had never even been away. I just went up to my bedroom, got into bed and closed my eyes, I didn't care if they never opened again.

May 2002

Steve and I had a really big argument today he said that he just couldn't cope with my depression anymore, we often have fall outs about this as Steve finds it really hard to deal with, but today was different he really meant it, he said that he thought we should break up. I feel I knew this was coming as I have been really bad lately but it didn't make it any easier. I went home and grabbed a bottle of red wine I found downstairs and took it up to my bedroom along with a glass. I smashed the glass on my dressing table and I grabbed one of the pieces. I stripped down to my underwear and started drinking the wine. I kept thinking that I didn't want to lose Steve. He is the best thing that has ever happened to me and it is all my fault if he leaves me.

I started scratching my thigh with the glass until it started to bleed when there were no more spaces on that thigh I started on the other, then my stomach then the rest of my legs each time I cut I would wait a couple of seconds then it would bleed. I blocked out the pain with the wine. I must have cut myself over two hundred times today, I hate what I do but I have to, because it is the only way I can cope with everything that is

going on inside my head.

Lonely

Lonely days

Lonely nights

Lonely heart

Lonely soul

Lonely smile

Lonely tears

Lonely life

There's no place like alone.

Hate

I hate the way I live a lie
I hate the way I have to cry.

I hate the waking up every day
Just to realise it hasn't gone away.

I hate the feeling of being alone
No one there on the end of the phone.

I hate the way no one knows the real me
They only see what they want to see

I hate the constant struggle just to get
     by
I hate the feeling of wanting to die

But above all else and without a doubt
It's me I hate, both inside and out.

Fake smiles

I've got a talent that I use every day
It's called faking a smile and saying
     things are okay.

I've perfected it to a tee over the years
They see all the smiles but I hide all the
     tears.

I wake in the morning and downstairs I
     go
To start my daily act and put on my
     show.

My pale skin is covered with powder so
     deep
And my shadows are hidden from the
     lack of sleep.

Lipstick and blusher, I've now finished
     my task
I look into the mirror at my much
     needed mask.

With a bit of makeup I can face the
       outside
No one could guess that inside I've died.

I smile at people as I go on my way
No one will question how I feel today.

She's happy with life that's plain to see
But that's just the person I dream to be.

No one sees the real me as I'm living
       this lie
They all smile at me as they walk on by.

Everything is great in my life, I'm so
       happy today
No questions are asked, it's easier that
       way.

But this act is slowly killing me inside
With every smile I show, it covers a tear
       I hide.

I wish I could just be myself and not
        give a damn
But who would really love me for the
        person that I really am ?

In Your Eyes

You're like me, you wear a mask too
But I can tell by your eyes when I look
    at you
Eyes never lie they say how you feel
You can't hide your eyes, what I see is
    real
You smile at me and say things are okay
But your eyes tell me what your voice
    cannot say
Disappointment rings out as you look
    straight through me
You dream of the person you want me
    to be
You can't understand why I feel as I do
You choose to ignore it, that's easier for
    you
You pretend not to see how I'm feeling
    inside
The fact I have an illness you choose to
    hide
I know you don't like me, that's plain to
    see

But why put on an act every time you
  see me?
Does it make you feel better if you're
  nice to my face?
But I've heard what you've said and no
  smile can erase
You hate the fact I've got depression,
  well I do too
I don't need your nasty comments, but
  support from you
I don't expect you to understand what's
  going on in my head
I've heard how you've judged me in the
  things you have said
Would you treat me this way if my
  illness you could see?
There's a person inside, she's called me
I have feelings and hopes. Of none you
  care
I have dreams and emotions that you
  don't want to share.

You're there always

You're there when I wake
You're there when I sleep
You're there when I sigh
You're there when I eat
You're there when I cry
Which I often do
You're there when I smile
To remind me not to.

Broken glass

I look at the floor to see
The broken glass shining against the
    light
I choose a piece which looks the best
And I hold it very tight

I then begin to shake and cry
As I study it very close
I look at every edge and angle
To find out which will hurt the most

I then begin to cut my stomach
Thighs, legs and arm
At this point I don't feel any pain
Just a sense of calm

I do this when the hurt inside
Gets to much to cope
It's my way of dealing with things.
It's my only hope.

I wish...

I wish I could laugh with those who
    laugh

I wish I could sing with those who sing

I wish I could dance with those who
    dance

I wish I could smile with those who
    smile

I wish I could live like those who live

I wish...

Portrait of hate

Sometimes it's hard to show you
Just how I really feel
Words don't seem to ever explain
So I hope this picture will.

They say a picture paints a thousand
      words
I'm hoping this is true
Because there is so much inside my
      head
 I just need to say to you.

I thought I'd do a portrait
A portrait of my life
To capture all my thoughts and fears
unhappiness and my strife.

I start by grabbing my canvas
Which is always by my side
I just have to pick what part to paint
That's never too hard to decide.

I then reach to find my tools
And lay them out upon the floor
I don't have much equipment, just the
      one
I find I don't need any more.

I don't use a paintbrush
But a razor blade instead
I don't paint in many colours
Just the one, which is red.

I always do my paintings from the heart
When words are hard to find
It's my way of living
in this messed up world of mine

My paintings don't have much structure
And they're never done with care
A few straight lines or maybe some
      curves
And some really deep ones here and
      there

Sometimes I paint over old paintings
Where the lines are now all raised

Some have been there years or months
Others, just days

After a while the red paint drips
And mimics the tears I've cried
The picture is now mixed together into
        a mess
Which is how I feel inside

I don't think you'll like my painting
Because it'll show you how I feel
 Before with just words you can block
        them out
But this you can't, you can see it, it's
        real

21st November 2005

It's been a week since I walked out of work and my head is now even more of a mess. I have spent the last seven days trying to work out what happened to me. Did I have some sort of breakdown? I just don't know. I have been to see my doctor and he has signed me off of work for four weeks. As each day goes by I am finding things harder to cope with and everything I used to do without trouble is taking more and more effort.

<u>29th November 2005</u>

I spent the whole day today in my pyjamas. I just couldn't push myself enough to get dressed. I can't explain the feeling but in a way it's like being in a straight jacket, no matter how much I want to do something I just can't physically move. There were cups and plates on the side from last night's dinner but how ever much I told myself that I needed to wash them up I just couldn't do it. I feel so frustrated and angry with myself.

WHAT'S WRONG WITH ME ! ! ! ! ! !

<u>19th December 2005</u>

It will soon be Christmas. I have put the decorations up for Steve's sake because if it was up to me I wouldn't have bothered. I just don't feel like it this year. Usually Christmas is my favourite time of the year and for the past ten years with depression I have always been able to push the sad feelings to the back of my mind and enjoy Christmas but this year is different. It feels as if I have pushed so much to the back of my mind that there is no more room. I'm trying so hard to be happy for Steve because I don't want to spoil it for him but it feels that I have nothing left inside to give anymore. The doctor

gave me another sick note for four more weeks

today.

I dream...

I dream of the day when I wake to find

No hurt in my heart

And no pain in my mind

Day in, day out

The curtains are drawn, no sunlight to
    see
The doors are all locked; I don't want
    anyone to see me

The phone rings out, but I don't pick up
    the receiver
The door bell goes but I don't answer
    that either

My pyjamas I wear all day and night
Too tired to try, too tired to fight

The TV's on loud to block out my mind
I stare at the screen, reality to find

I rock back and forth as I try to
    comprehend
This world that I live in with no
    beginning or end

My hair hangs dirty, my face is a mess

But who will ever see, no need to
impress

I sit for hour upon hour powerless to
move
My meaning in this world, unable to
prove

My shadow

Depression is my shadow
It never leaves my side
Wherever I go, wherever I turn
There's never anywhere to hide.
It's with me day and night
And watches me when I cry
It has so much control of me
It makes me want to die.
I've tried to run away from it
And pretend it's gone away
But it surrounds me with it's darkness
And tells me it's here to stay.
It tells me I should hate myself
Because everyone hates me too
It tells me I'd be better off dead
That would be the best thing I could do.
It tells me no one loves me
And no one really cares
They all think I'm a failure
Am I blind not to see their stares.
It tells me no one will save me
No one really wants me around

No one would ever miss me
When I'm buried in the ground.
It tells me I am useless
And a total waste of space
That I will never be happy
Reality I need to face.
And when I'm alone
In the middle of the night
Crying on my pillow
It holds me so tight.
It tells me it can help me
That it's my only friend
That all this pain and misery
it can help me to end.
It makes me go downstairs
And get a knife out of the drawer
It tells me I'm too weak
That I can't carry on any more.
We go back upstairs
I take the knife to my skin
It tells me it'll soon be over
With a gentle nudge and a grin.
It tells me to cut deeper
To cut all the pain away
That this is my only hope

That I need to die today.
But I just can't do it
I throw the knife upon the floor
I close my eyes so tight
And my shadow walks to the door.
But before it goes
With a smile it turns to say
Don't worry I'm not leaving you
I'm never going away.

<u>28th January 2006</u>

I have been really bad today, I just don't want to go on anymore. I've really had enough of constantly battling with myself.

And I just feel like giving up. Today all I have done is sit in my pyjamas on the settee and rock back and fourth crying. I went back to bed this afternoon because when I am asleep that is the only time I get a break from my mind but I just wish I would never wake up again.

5th February 2006

I went to occupational health today in work, because I have been off sick for so long they wanted to see me. I was lucky because Steve was off of work today so he took me. I haven't been out on my own for about twelve weeks. The thought of doing so makes me feel physically sick. I hate the way I feel like a prisoner in my own home but I'm not ready yet to take that step back into the outside world. Hopefully one day.

4th April 2006

Today was a big day for me, I handed my notice in at work and it broke my heart. Although I feel much better in myself the past five months have taken a lot out of me including my self-confidence and self esteem which are both rock bottom. Although I would love nothing more than to walk back through those doors that I walked out of all those months ago I know I'm not strong enough to do so. The thought of being around all those people again which I used to love to be, and the thought of helping the new mothers with their babies which used to bring me so much happiness, no matter how much I desperately wanted to go back to how things used to be the thought of going through those doors again filled me with utter dread so giving in my notice was really my only option. I didn't want to face the prospect of going back down again so in a way it was a coward's way out and I feel such a failure for doing so.

Why me?

I wake to another day of darkness
A struggle just to live
The smallest task feels enormous
I have nothing left to give

Today is the same as yesterday
With the world just passing me by
I look out of my window
With a tear in my eye

I wish people could understand
Just how I felt inside
To everyone I'm just normal
Because my feelings I have to hide

Why do I have to have this illness?
Why did it pick me?
I so much just want to be happy
And be released of this misery.

<u>What do you think ?</u>

Do you think this is how I want to live
    my life ?
running away from the person I've
    become ?

Do you think this is how I dreamed my
    life would turn out
when I was a little girl ?

Do you think I enjoy cutting myself ?
and making myself bleed ?

Do you think I want to stay locked up in
    my house
too scared of the outside world ?

Do you think I like to cry day and night
and have to fake my smiles ?

Do you think I do this all for attention ?
Do you really think that little of me ?

I'm fine

I often meet people
And they sometimes say
Why so down?
What's gone wrong today?
How do I explain how I'm feeling
    inside?
The feeling of emptiness and the
    heartache I hide?
How can I tell them what's wrong with
    my head?
I can't...
So I smile sweetly and say, "I'm fine,"
    instead.

Pebbles on the beach

I feel like a pebble
That's lost within the sea
I scream for a helping hand
For someone to rescue me

But my cries are lost
With the sound of the waves
As they crash on the shoreline
Maybe I can't be saved

The sway of the tide
Brings me closer to shore
As it pushes me to safety
But then drags me out once more

It's like a cruel game
That it plays with me
Showing me a glimpse of hope
Before I'm dragged out to sea

I see all the other pebbles
Fighting the same fight
We look to the shore
Happiness is in sight

It's not a fair match
As I resist the sea
I feel so small and useless
As it opens and swallows me

But I fight back
With every thing inside
As the battle commences
Between me and the tide

I've made it! I'm safe
I feel the warmth of the sun
I'm a bit scratched and battered
But who cares, I've won!

But then along comes someone
Who picks me up high
They hold me so tight
I let out a cry

They swing their arm back
And toss me up high
A smile fills my face
As I fly through the sky

But as I look down
My smile disappears
As I see the deep ocean
My eyes fill with tears

I'm back here again
In this dark empty place
As I sink deeper and deeper
And disappear without a trace.

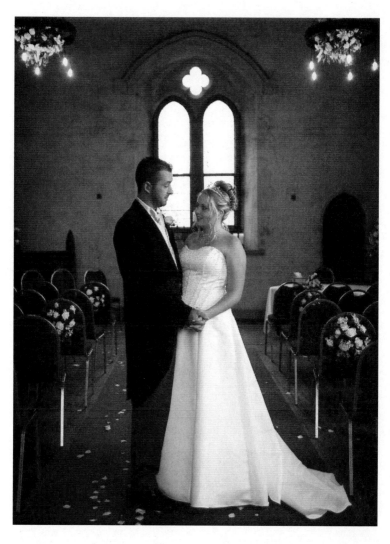

Our wedding day 24th July 2005

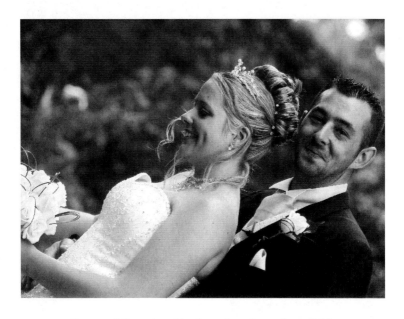

Our wedding day (the happiest day of my life).

And finally...

I'd like to end by saying thank you for taking the time to read my book I just hope I have managed to help you in some way, if you are going through the same situation you may feel alone, this was one of my biggest feelings, loneliness, I felt that no one understood me but then I came to realise, how could anyone really understand what is going on inside someone else's head? Only one person knows truly how you feel and that is yourself. So once you have come to terms with your feelings and understand that depression is not your fault, it is in fact an illness, the next stage is to tell others. You will probably be met by a very mixed response, some may be shocked, others supportive, some will be evasive and others may also be unkind. But whatever you come across just remember that with admitting you have a problem first to yourself, then to others you will be taking the first steps up the ladder to getting better. You may have already taken those steps with telling people and you may feel no better. If this is the case I would personally like to encourage you to see your GP and ask for more help, you might need medication, you might need counselling or you may need both but whatever you need don't feel like a failure like I felt because you are not, all you are is someone who is a bit stuck at the moment and you need a little bit of help to get free again. I have come such a long way since I reached my lowest point and that is what I think of whenever I feel down. I'm not going to lie to you and tell you that I am all better now, because I'm not, there are times when I feel that I could quite easily fall right back down again. What's changed over the last twelve years is I have come to accept depression and most of all I have come to accept me and with excepting me for who I am I'm no longer scared or ashamed with showing or saying how I feel and that in turn has made depression so much easier to deal with. I know this is not the happy ending for me, I know this battle between me and IT will carry on for maybe the rest of my life. But I can hand on heart say I will never let it drag me down that far again. If depression has given me anything positive it has given me strength, strength to fight for the happy life that used to be only in my dreams but is now starting to become reality.

Please don't do it alone

All my love

Emma

X X X

My World...

Welcome to my world
In this world you exist on your own
Everything that ever goes wrong in it, is your fault
Everything that you dream about will never happen
They just remain dreams that will gradually fade
away
There's never sunshine, just night time
There's never happy times, just sad times
You feel like you are in a bubble
But however much you try, it will never burst
You don't live life, you endure it
It's a nightmare but there's no way of waking from
it
Do you want to be in my world?
No?
I didn't think so.

What, Why, When

What is wrong with me?
I ask that question every day
Why can't I just get better?
Why can't depression just go away?
Why can't I wake up in the morning
And everything will be alright?
Why can't I find in my tunnel
The end with the brilliant light?
Why can't I just snap out of it?
And for once be happy today
Why can't I just get better?
Why can't depression just go away?
Why am I so lost in my own world?
Too scared to venture outside
Why is my head filled with mixed feelings?
Most of which I have to hide
How long will this go on for?
How many more years will I feel this way?
When will I get better?
When will depression just go away?

Since my book has gone to publish I can happily say that I have now found part-time work in a shop. I know previously I said that I felt that I would never work again but I have now proved myself wrong and I am very proud of this achievement. The first steps were definitely the hardest, facing my biggest fears head on and there were times when I was so scared of the prospect of going back to work that I felt it would be so much easier to just forget about the whole idea, but then I asked myself what I wanted out of my life, did I want my life to carry on the way it was or was I prepared to push myself to my absolute limits and finally break this unhappy cycle that I was just existing in, so with that in mind I pushed myself harder than I had ever done before and with each new day I began to relax and for once actually started to enjoy this new person inside, someone that I had lost a long, long time ago, I found Emma and you know what? I actually quite like her!

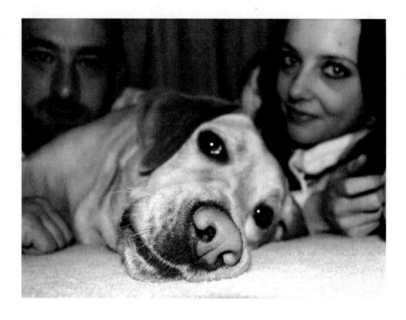

Steve, me and Holly now.